Thirty Breathing Exercises
to Help Children to Calm and Focus

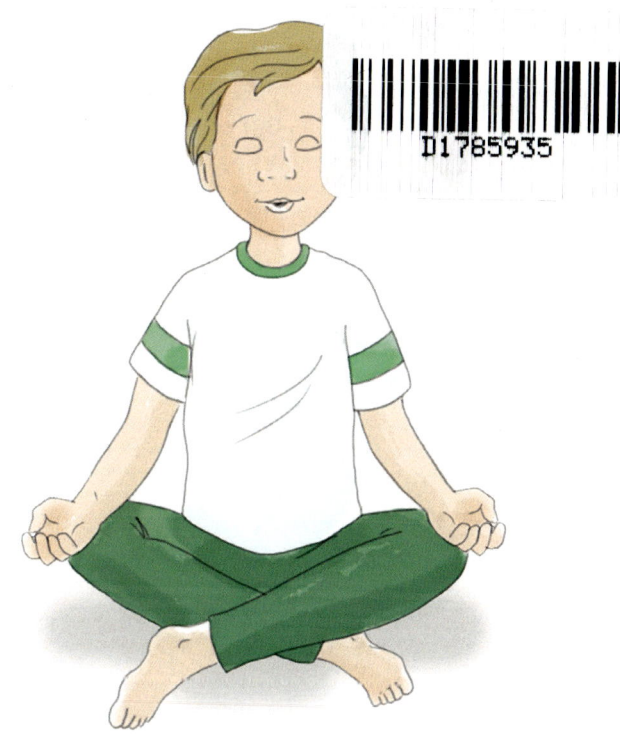

Breathing Exercises
FOR KIDS

Written by Giselle Shardlow
www.KidsYogaStories.com

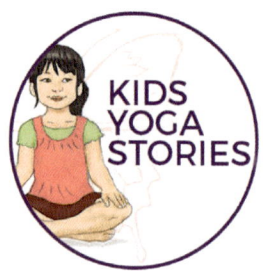

www.KidsYogaStories.com

Copyright © 2018 by Giselle Shardlow
Cover and breath illustrations by Valerie Bouthyette
All images © 2018 Giselle Shardlow

All rights reserved. No part of this book may be reproduced in any form by any electronic or mechanical means, including photocopying, recording, or information storage and retrieval without written permission from the author. The author, illustrator, and publisher accept no responsibility or liability for any injuries or losses that may result from practicing the breathing techniques outlined in this book. Please ensure your own safety and the safety of the children.

ISBN: 978-1-943648-33-7

Kids Yoga Stories
Boston, MA
www.kidsyogastories.com
www.amazon.com/author/giselleshardlow

Email us at info@kidsyogastories.com.

What do you think? Let us know what you think
of *Breathing Exercises for Kids* at feedback@kidsyogastories.com.

Index

Alternate Nostril Breathing	2
Back-to-Back Breathing	4
Balloon Breath	6
Bee Breath	8
Bunny Breath	10
Candle Breath	12
Cooling Breath	14
Count Down to Calm	16
Deep Belly Breath	18
Eagle Breath	20
Extended Exhale	22
Feather Breath	24
Figure Eight Breath	26
Flower Breath	28
Flying Bird Breath	30
Hoberman Breath	32
Lion's Breath	34
Loving-Kindness Breath	36
Mindful Breathing	38
Ocean Breath	40
Pompom Breath	42
Power Breath	44
Rubbing Hands Breath	46
Shoulder Breath	48
Snake Breath	50
Take 5 Breath	52
Three Deep Breaths	54
Truck Driver Breath	56
Volcano Breath	58
Woodchopper Breath	60
Breathing Exercise Games	63

Welcome to Breathing Exercises for Kids

Are you looking for a collection of easy breathing techniques to practice with your children?

This book is for primary school teachers, kids yoga teachers, parents, caregivers, health practitioners, and recreation staff looking for simple, convenient ways to add breathing exercises into their curriculum, classes, or home life.

Tips to make your breathing exercise experience as successful as possible:

- Breathing techniques can be practiced in various positions, such as sitting comfortably cross-legged on the ground, sitting in a chair, sitting on your heels in Hero Pose, or lying flat on your back in Resting Pose.

- Don't worry if you don't get the breathing technique the first time. Go easy on yourself and keep practicing. Think of this as a lifelong practice that evolves over time.

- The most important part is to become aware of your breathing. Feel the rise and fall of your breath and how your breathing affects your body.

- These breathing techniques are meant to inspire you with ideas, so feel free to encourage the children's imagination and creativity.

- On each exhale, work on releasing stress and tension from your mind and body.

- The number of breaths you practice will depend on the age, energy levels, and needs of your children. Tune into your children, and you'll know what is best for them.

- Familiarize yourself with the breathing technique before introducing it to your children.

- Focus on playing around with these breathing techniques and keep it light-hearted and fun.

- Be engaging and enthusiastic as you try new breathing exercises together.

- Feel free to add your own props, music, relaxation stories, or songs to make the experience more meaningful for your children.

- Set up the environment beforehand so the children know what to expect by practicing these breathing exercises. Slow down, capture their attention, and help them focus.

- Practice specific breathing exercises that match your learning topic. For example, practice Flower Breath with your studies of spring.

- After repeating the breathing exercise a few times, open your eyes and come to breathing naturally. Feel the effects of the breath.

Get children using their breath to help them to calm and focus with these quick and easy breathing techniques!

Breathing Exercises
FOR KIDS

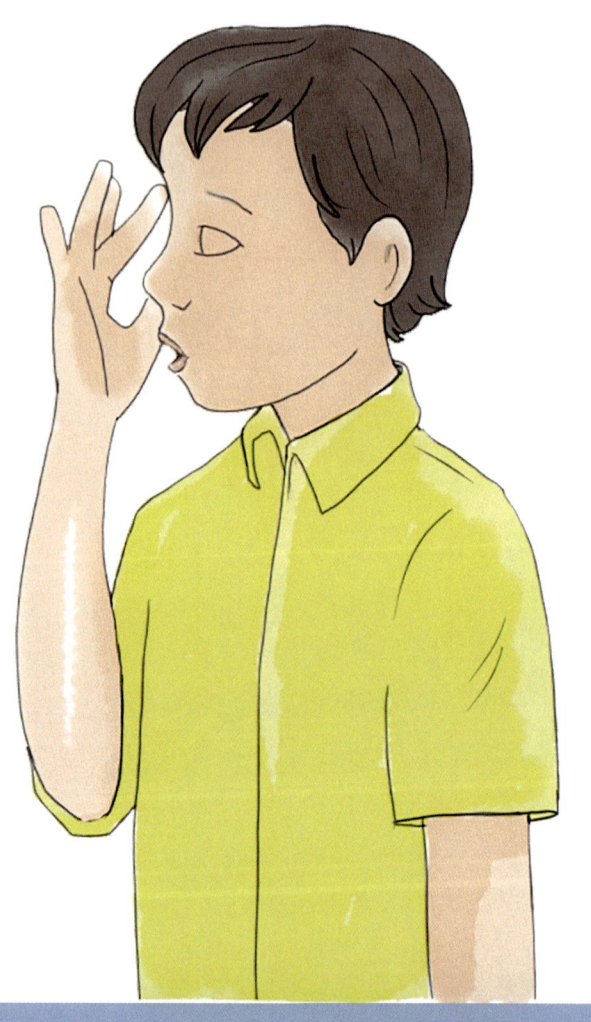

Alternate Nostril Breathing

Alternate Nostril Breathing

Place your middle finger of your right hand on your forehead between your eyebrows (third eye center). Close your right nostril gently with your right thumb and inhale slowly through your left nostril. Pause at the top of your inhale and release your right thumb. Close your left nostril gently with your ring finger and exhale slowly through your right nostril. Pause at the bottom of your exhale then inhale through your right nostril. Pause at the top of the inhale, release your ring finger, close your right nostril with your thumb, and exhale through your left nostril. Repeat these steps at least four times.

> VARIATION: Younger children might find it easier to use their pointer finger to close their nostrils.

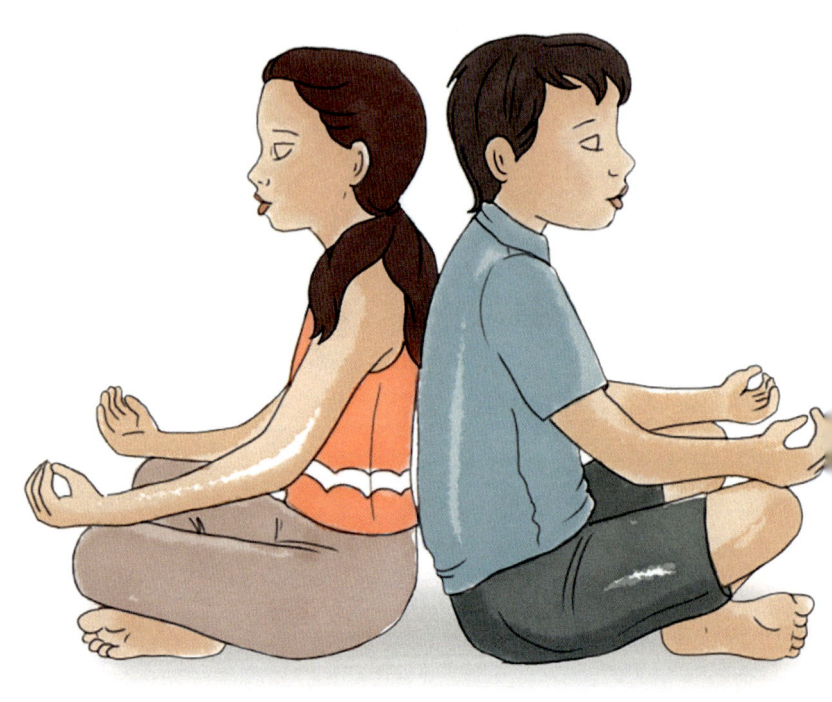

Back-to-Back Breathing

Back-to-Back Breathing

Pick a partner and sit back-to-back on the floor in a cross-legged position. Take a moment to ensure that your spines are straight and that you are comfortably touching each other's backs. Place your palms on your knees. When you're both ready, take in a deep inhale for three counts, then exhale deeply together for three counts. Repeat this three-count inhale and three-count exhale, focusing on keeping your breath rhythm together. Feel the breath movement on your partner's back. Close your eyes, if that's comfortable.

> VARIATION: Have one person sit on the other person's lap, close to their chest, to feel the rise and fall of their breath.

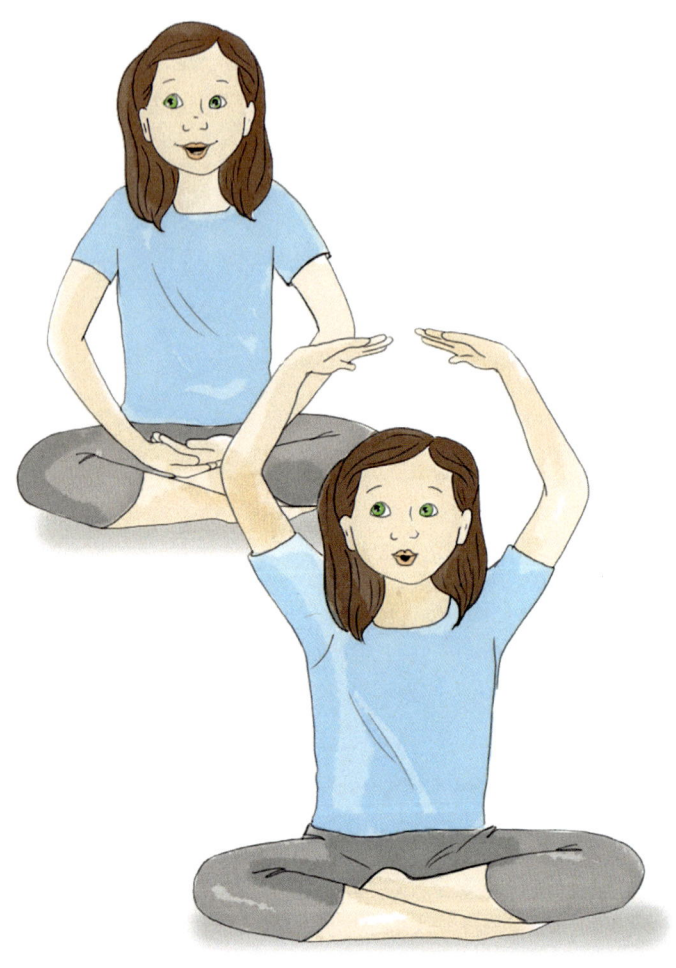

Balloon Breath

Balloon Breath

Take a deep breath in for three counts while raising your arms to form the shape of a balloon. With your lips closed, exhale through your nose for three counts while taking your hands back to rest on your knees. Feel the rise and fall of your chest and belly as you continue to raise and lower your arms like a balloon inflating and deflating.

> IMAGINE: Being a hot air balloon in the middle of a meadow.

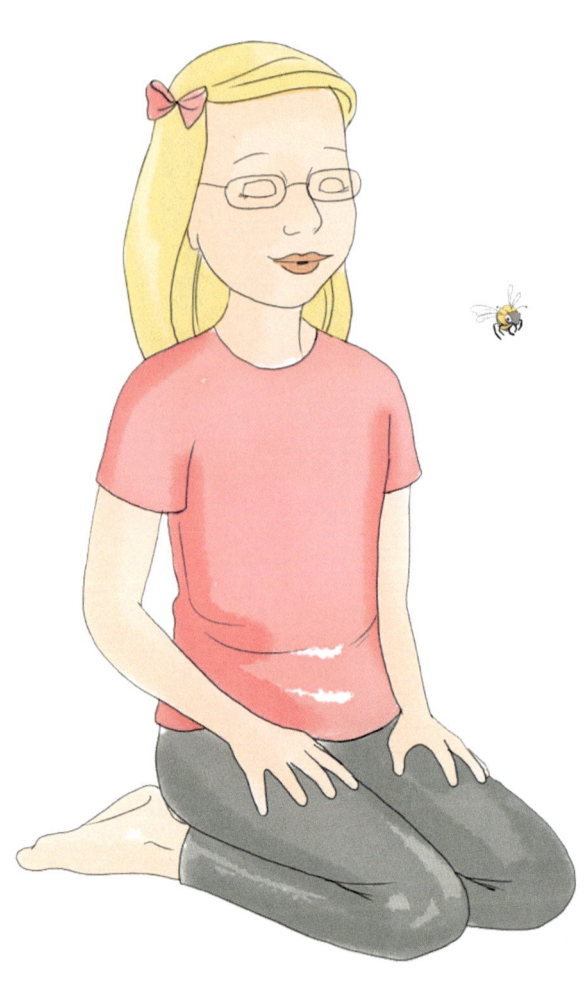

Bee Breath

Bee Breath

As you exhale, keep your mouth closed and make a long "mmm" sound, pretending to buzz like a bee around the garden. Then inhale through your nose, keeping your mouth closed. Repeat the bee-humming sound as you exhale. Close your eyes and continue in this way for a few minutes or as long as it feels comfortable. You could also cup your hands over your ears to intensify the "mmm" sound.

VARIATION: Make the sound of a train whistle.

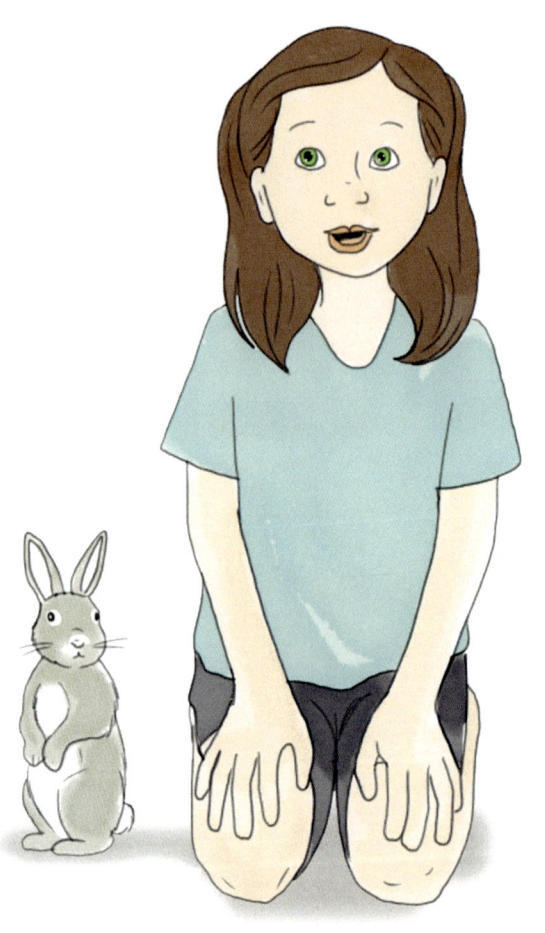

Bunny Breath

Bunny Breath

Come to sitting on your heels in Hero Pose, pretending to be a bunny. Sniff for food by taking three to five short inhales, pause, then exhale slowly—all with a closed mouth, if possible. Repeat a few times.

> VARIATIONS: Imagine sniffing spring flowers, freshly baked cookies, or a candy store.

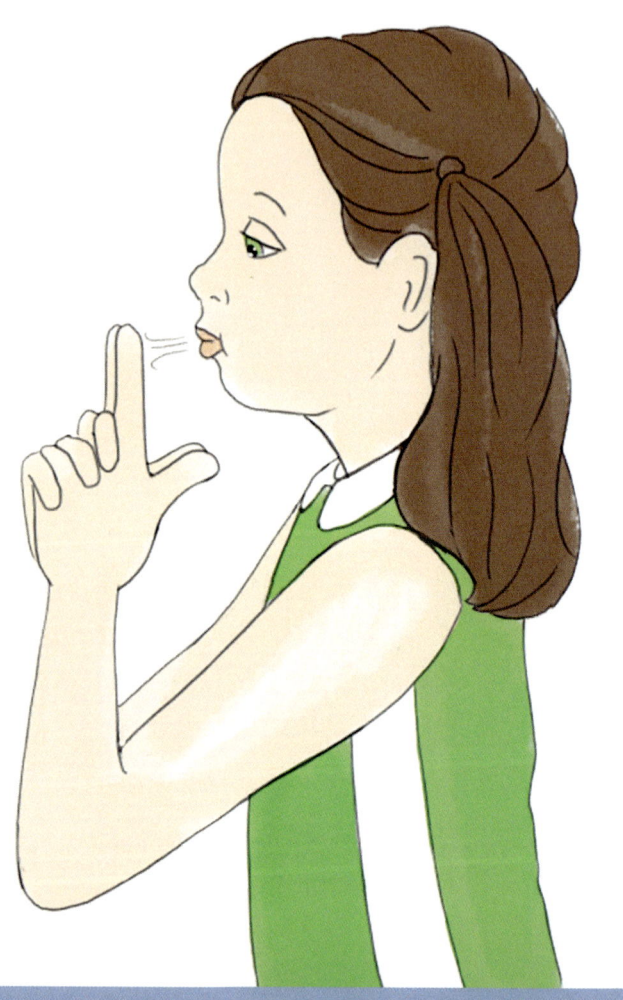

Candle Breath

Candle Breath

Clasp your fingers together and extended your pointer fingers up like a steeple. Pretending it's a candle, bring your steepled hands in front of your mouth. Take a deep breath in through your nose then pretend to blow out your candle. Close your eyes, if that's comfortable. Repeat a few times.

VARIATIONS: Blow a flower or pinwheel.

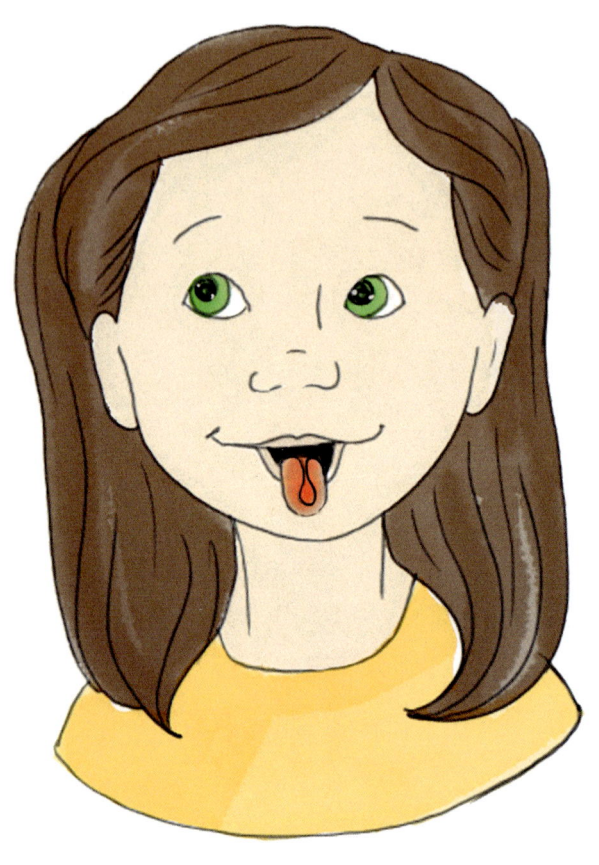

Cooling Breath

Cooling Breath

Take a few breaths to calm your mind and body. When you are ready, curl your tongue lengthwise, as if your tongue is a hot dog bun wrapping around a hot dog. Inhale gently through your mouth, feeling the breath cool your tongue. Then close your mouth and exhale through your nose. Repeat this a few times to get the hang of it then return to breathing normally.

> IMAGINE: Sucking a fruit smoothie through a straw on a hot summer day.

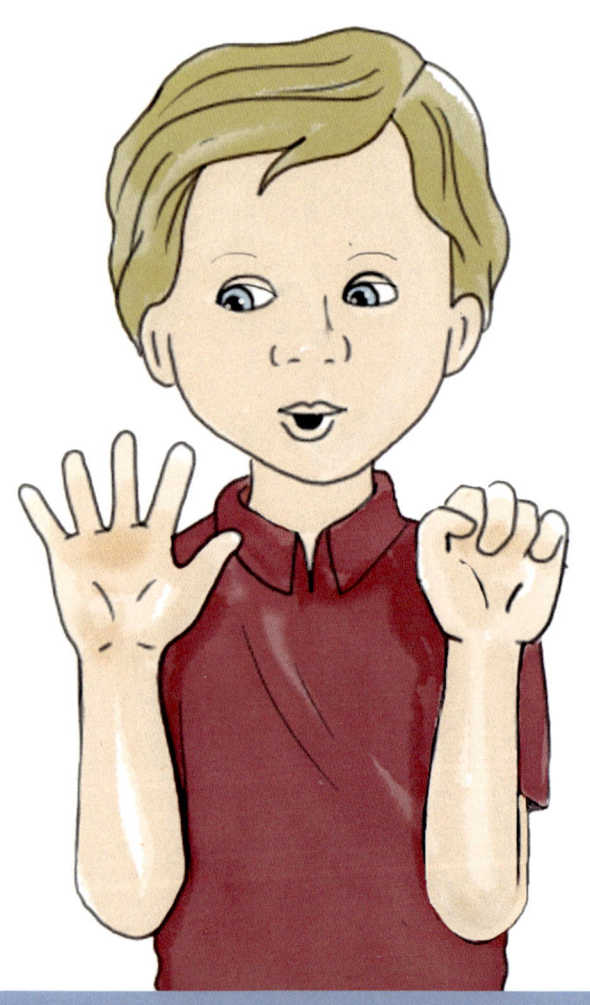

Count Down to Calm

Count Down to Calm

Take your right hand out in front of you, fingers spread. Take in a deep inhale, then exhale slowly while counting down from 5 to 1 and bringing a finger down for each count. Bring your thumb down; count "one." Bring your second finger down; count "two." Bring your middle finger down; count "three." Bring your ring finger down; count "four." Bring your pinky finger down; count "five." Then take a deep inhale for five counts while slowly spreading open your fingers. Repeat the steps a few times until you feel calm.

> IMAGINE: Your fingers are foxes and they go home to their den.

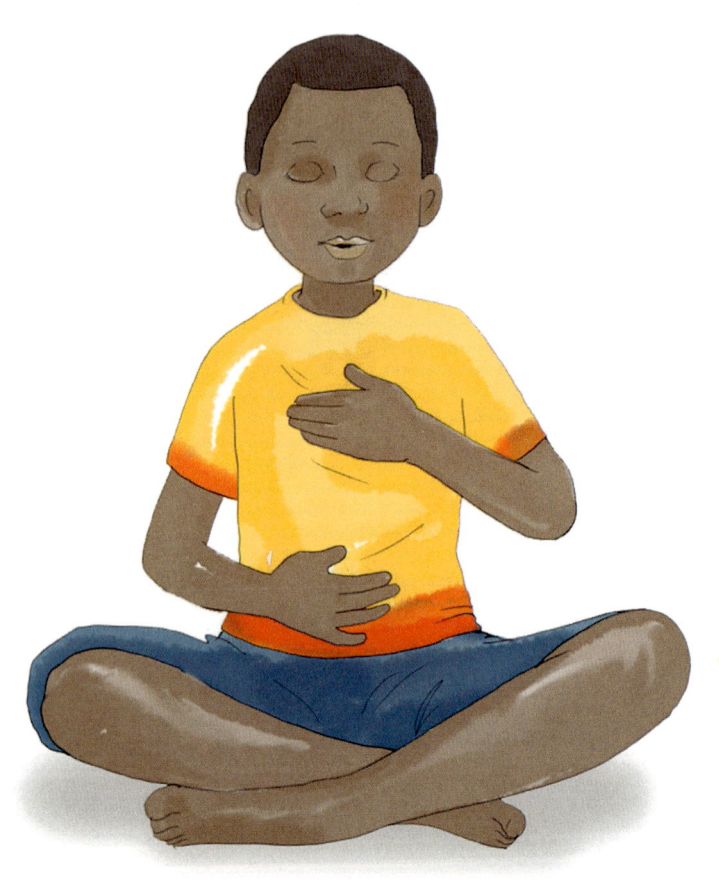

Deep Belly Breath

Deep Belly Breath

Place your right hand on your belly and your left hand on your chest. Take a deep breath in for four counts then exhale through your nose for four counts, with your lips closed. Feel the rise and fall of your chest and belly. If you're on your back, you could place an object, like a stuffed animal, on your stomach to help you feel (and see) the rise and fall of your belly. Do this deep belly breathing for a few minutes.

> IMAGINE: Different things you are grateful for during each inhale and exhale.

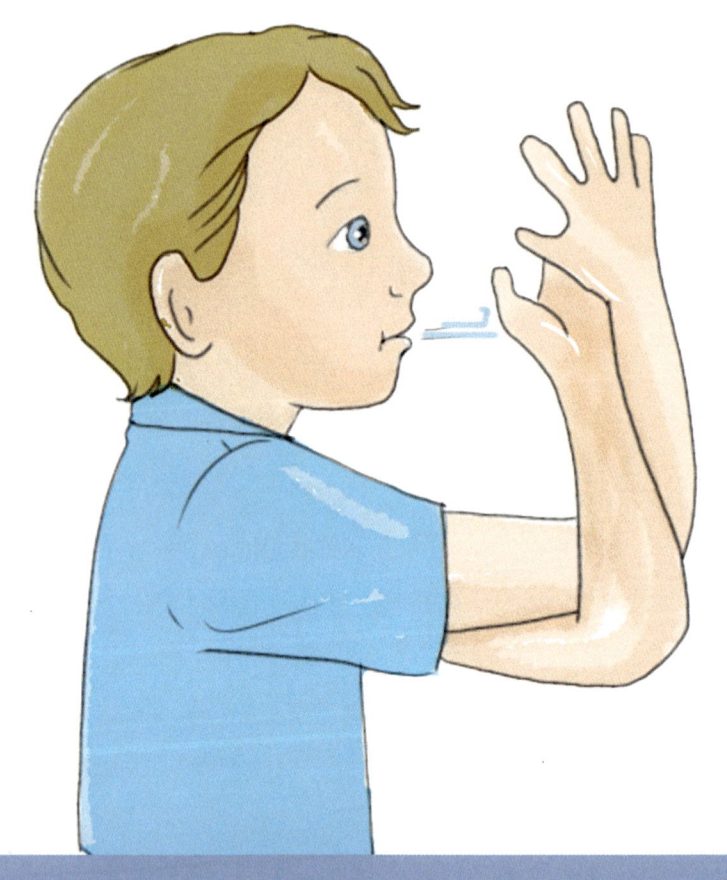

Eagle Breath

Eagle Breath

Create "eagle arms" by wrapping your right arm under your left arm, so your elbows are hooked together, and bring your palms together directly in front of your face. When you're ready, take a deep inhale, unwrap your arms, and switch sides with eagle arms so that your left elbow will be on the bottom. Exhale deeply and relax your shoulders. Repeat the steps by linking your movement to changing sides of your eagle arms.

> VARIATION: Instead of Eagle Arms, simply place your palms on opposite shoulders and touch your elbows together. Inhale, bringing your palms up to touch, then exhale, bringing your palms back down to the opposite shoulders.

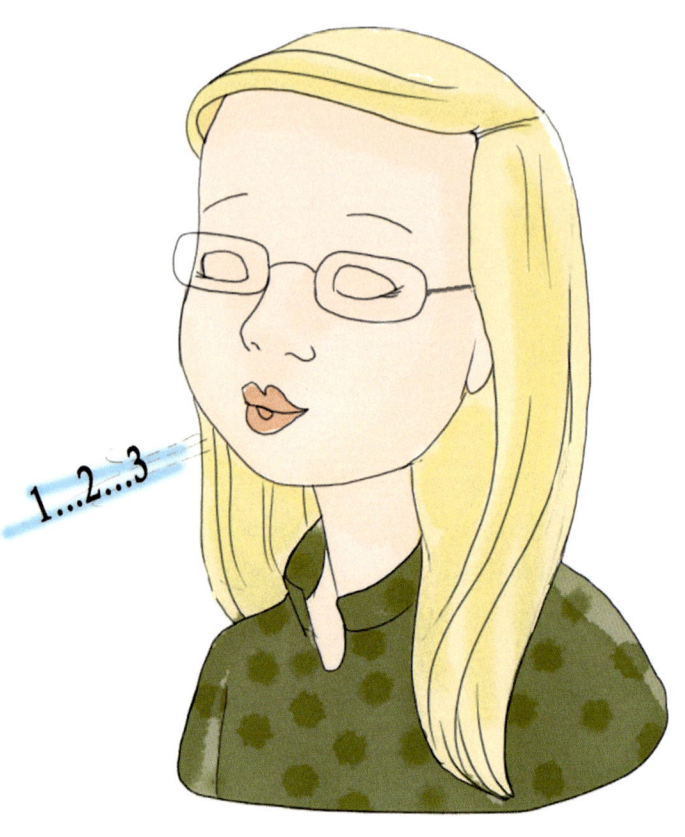

Extended Exhale

Extended Exhale

Take a deep inhale for three to five counts. Then exhale slowly for six to ten counts. Try to make your exhale twice as long as your inhale. Repeat a few times.

IMAGINE: Blowing bubbles or leaves.

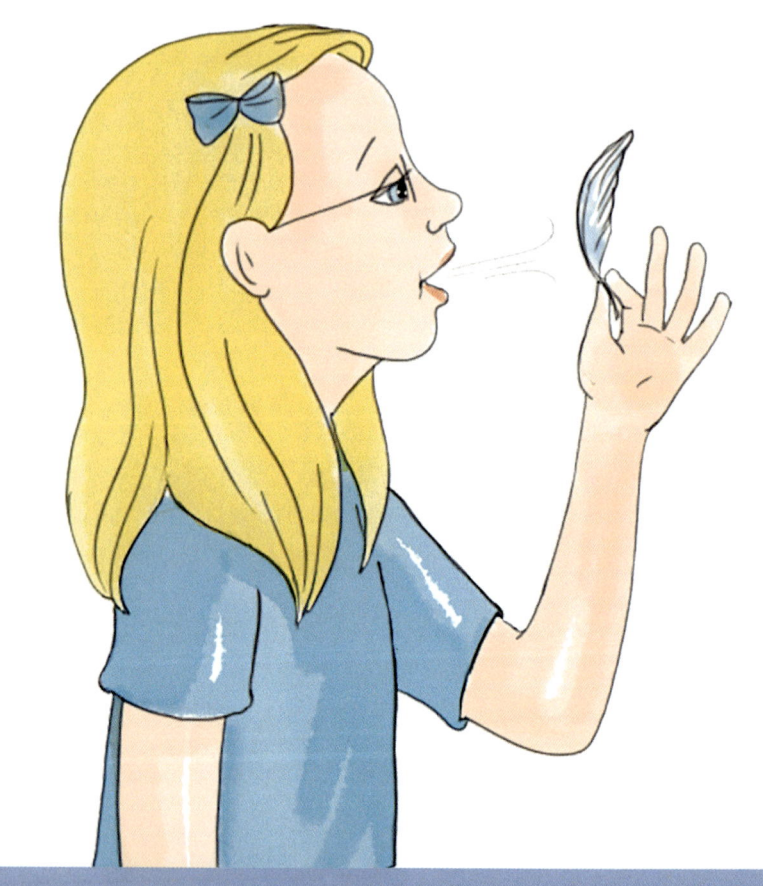

Feather Breath

Feather Breath

Hold a feather out in front of you. Take in a deep breath then blow the feather. Watch it flutter with your breath. Repeat a few times.

> VARIATIONS: Try using a pinwheel, scarf, or anything that would move with your breath.

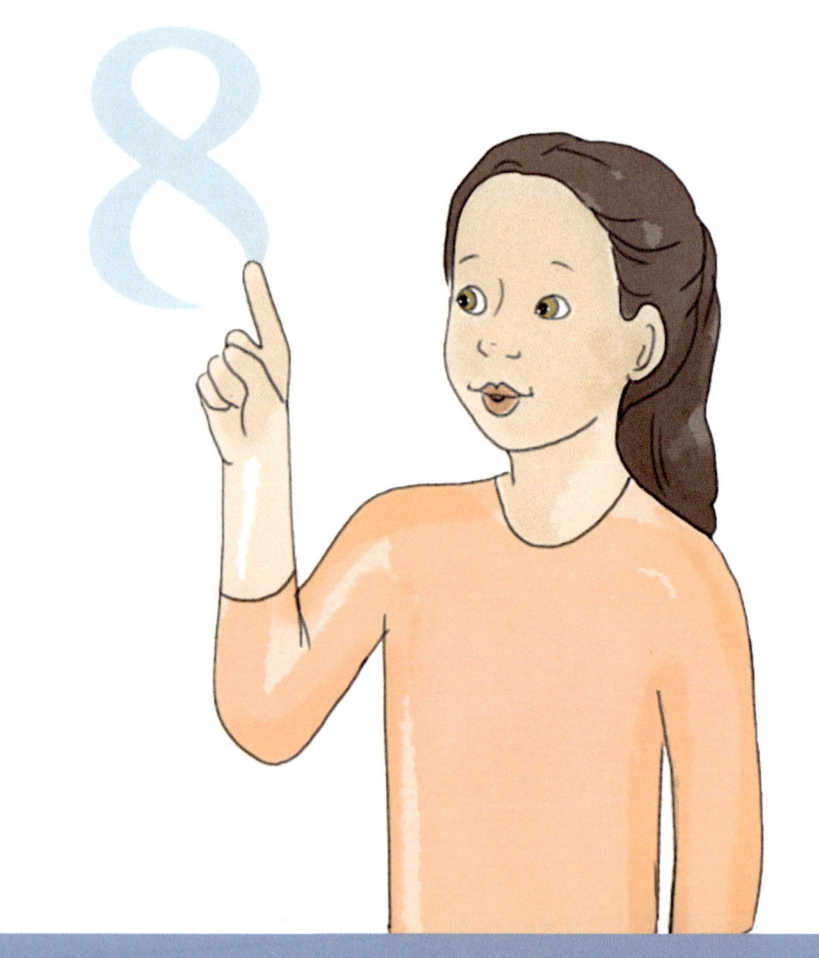

Figure Eight Breath

Figure Eight Breath

Take your pointer finger out in front of you. As you trace a figure "8" in the air, practice inhaling and exhaling deeply. Focus your eyes on your moving finger and feel your belly expand and contract with your deep belly breathing.

VARIATION: Trace a zero or any other shape.

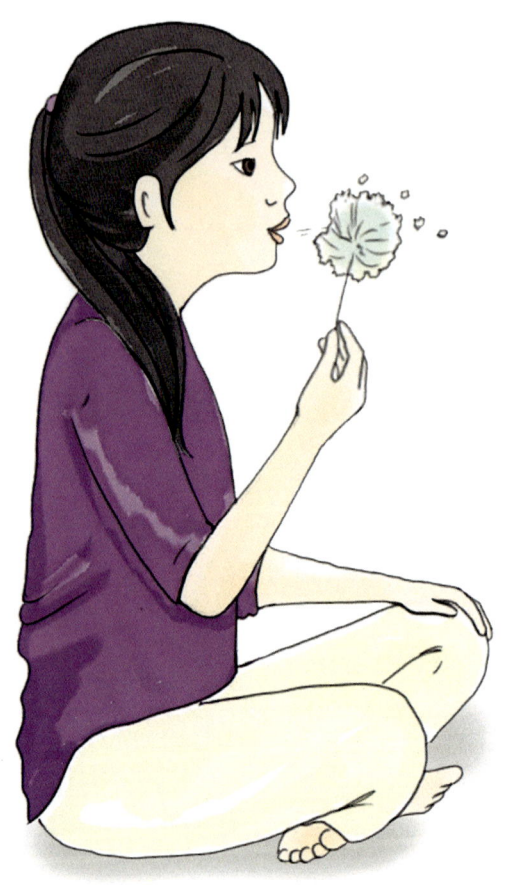

Flower Breath

Flower Breath

Imagine holding a flower. Imagine the color and smell of that flower. Then take in a deep breath through your nose, pretending to smell that flower. Then exhale through your mouth and pretend to blow the flower petals. Repeat the cycle of a strong inhale and gentle exhale for a couple of minutes, if possible. You could pretend to smell a different flower each time you inhale. You could also imagine yourself sitting in a meadow of fresh flowers.

VARIATION: Sniff and blow on hot chocolate.

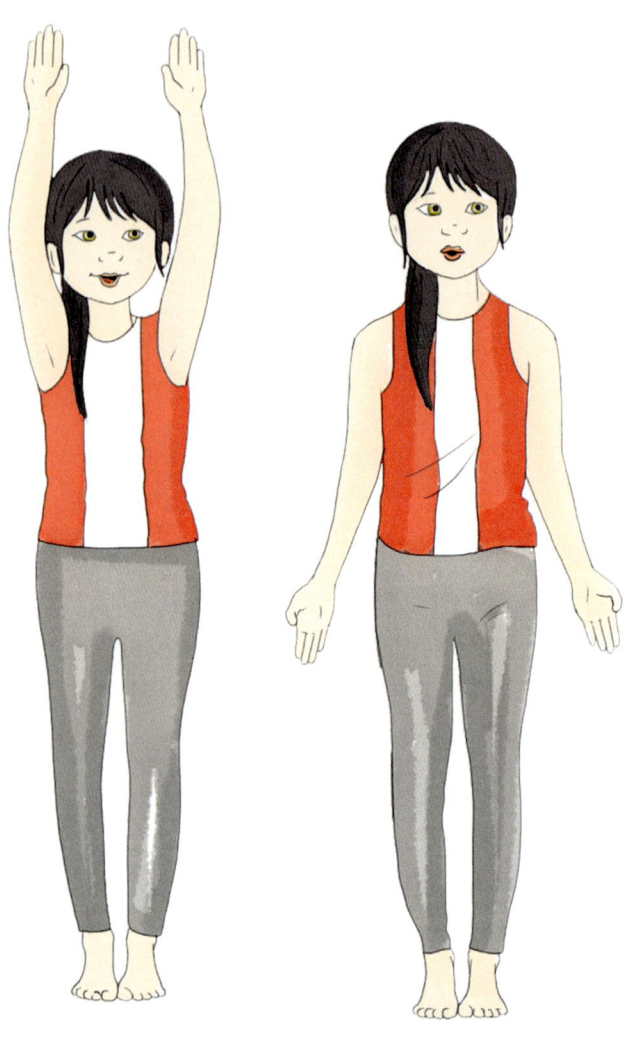

Flying Bird Breath

Flying Bird Breath

Standing in Mountain Pose, imagine being a bird flying through the sky. As you inhale, lift your arms over your head, touching your palms together. Then as you exhale, bring your arms back down to your sides, touching your palms to your outer thighs. Continue this flow for a few minutes, pretending to sync the movements of your body with the motion of flapping wings.

> VARIATION: Be a butterfly flapping its wings or a peacock opening its feathers.

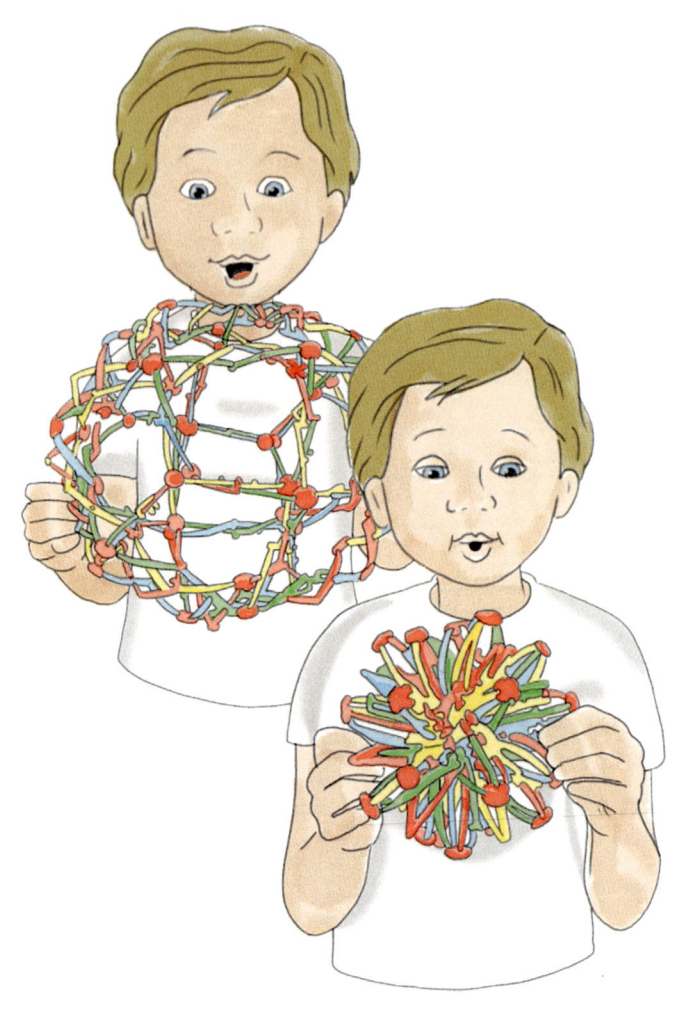

Hoberman Breath

Hoberman Breath

Bring your Hoberman sphere in front of your chest. Inhale slowly, expanding the Hoberman sphere to mimic your chest expanding with your deep breath. As you exhale slowly, make the Hoberman sphere smaller to mimic pushing the air from your lungs. Repeat this exercise a few times.

> IMAGINE: The Hoberman sphere is a balloon or a ball that you are blowing up.

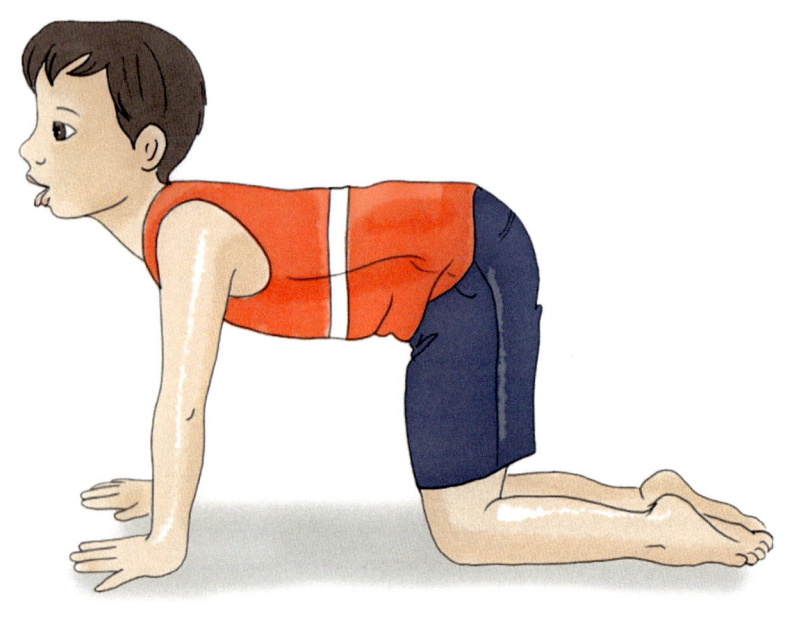

Lion's Breath

Lion's Breath

Come to an all-fours position (or Hero Pose). Take a deep breath in through your nose then look forward. As you exhale, open your mouth, stick out your tongue, and exhale audibly, making a "ha" sound. Repeat the steps, ending by exhaling through your mouth with your tongue out, pretending to be a lion. Repeat the lion's breath a few times while it feels comfortable then breathe naturally.

VARIATION: Be a dragon breathing fire.

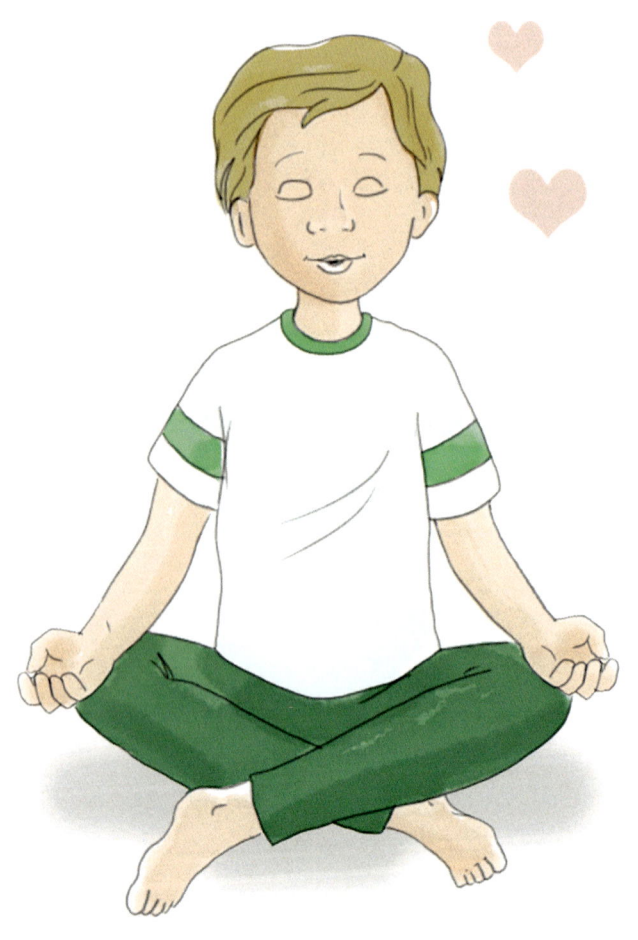

Loving-Kindness Breath

Loving-Kindness Breath

As you exhale, think of filling yourself with love. Imagine the color red enveloping your body as you inhale. On the next exhale, think of sending love and kindness to someone close to you. On the next exhale, send loving kindness to someone you're having a difficult relationship with. Then send love and kindness out to the world around you: the animals, the trees, your neighbors, and your community. Lastly, send out love and kindness to the world. Finish your loving kindness breath by coming back to breathing naturally. When you are ready, open your eyes.

IMAGINE: Sending love for Valentine's Day.

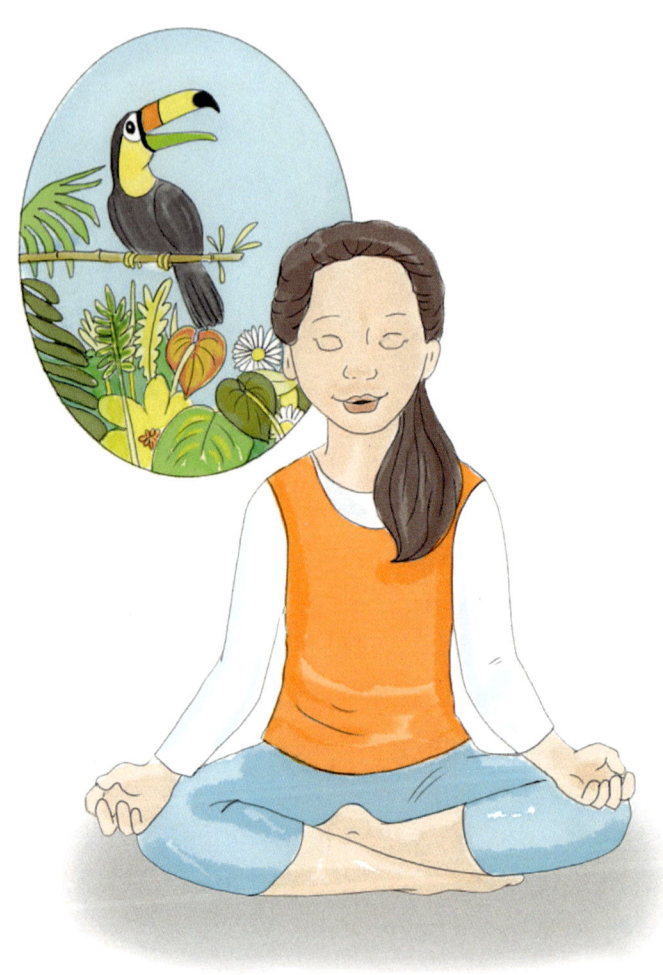

Mindful Breathing

Mindful Breathing

Take a few breaths to calm your mind and body. When you are ready, take a three-count inhale followed by a three-count exhale. Once you have the rhythm of your mindful breathing, start to imagine the sounds you might hear in the rainforest. Think of frogs croaking, birds singing, monkeys howling, snakes hissing, and rain falling. You could also play rainforest sounds in the background to help you imagine the rainforest. Imagine the smells of the rainforest and feel the humid heat on your body. Continue with this mindful breathing technique for a few minutes, as long as it feels comfortable to you.

> VARIATIONS: Pretend to be on the beach, in the woodlands, or in the desert.

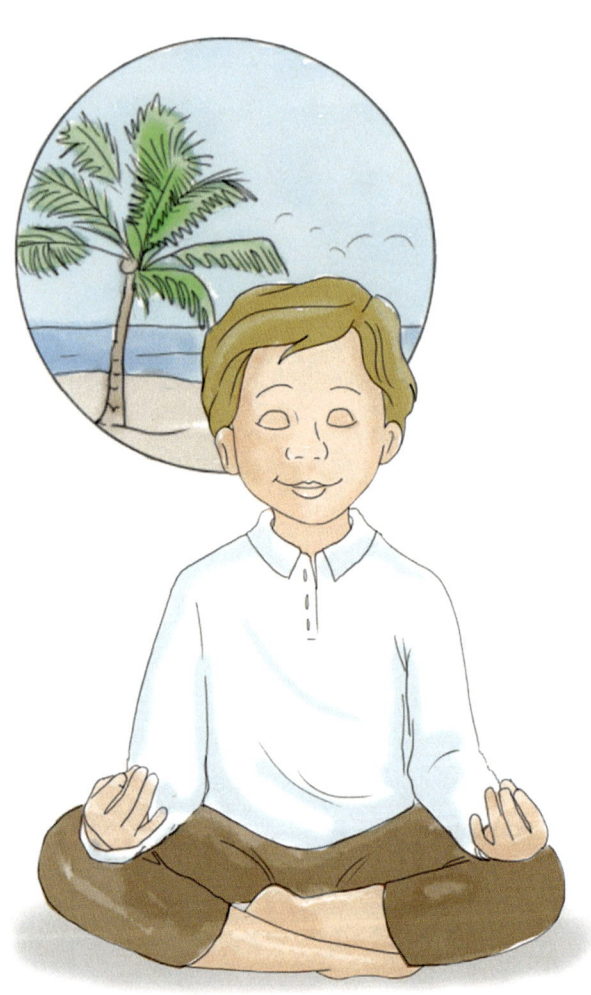

Ocean Breath

Ocean Breath

Breathe in and out through your nose with your mouth closed. As you exhale, make an audible sound in the back of your throat, like the sound of the ocean. Exhale audibly for a count of three, followed by an inhale for another count of three. Close your eyes and imagine sitting on the beach, listening to the waves crashing on the beach. Continue with this three-count breath for a few minutes.

> VARIATION: Hold your hand in front of your face and blow on your palm, making a "haa" sound as if you are fogging up a mirror.

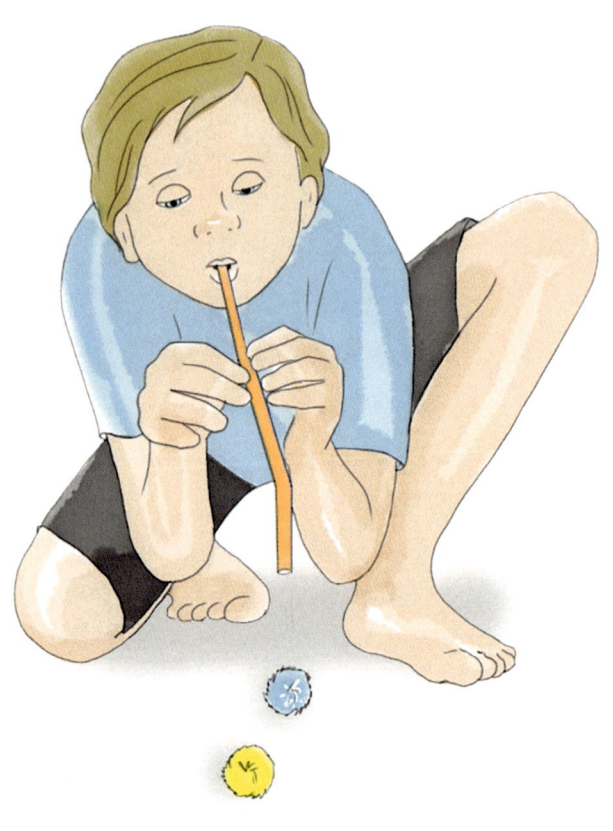

Pompom Breath

Pompom Breath

Place several cotton balls or pompoms on a table or on the floor. Use a straw to blow the pompoms around. Talk to the children about the effects of a gentle or hard breath.

> IMAGINE: Playing a soccer game and blow the pompoms between goal posts.

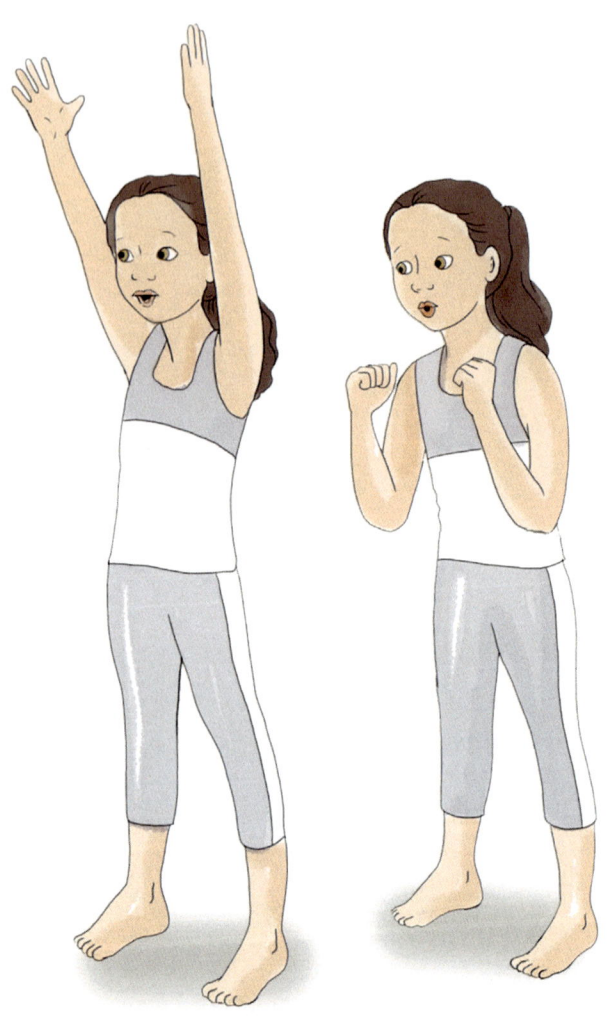

Power Breath

Power Breath

Clench your hands into fists above your head then exhale vigorously through your mouth, saying, "Ha!" At the same time, bring your fists quickly to your chest while tucking your elbows against your body. Think of pulling the power of the sun into your body through your chest. Repeat this breathing technique a few times to bring warmth to your body. You can also try it with one arm at a time.

> IMAGINE: Celebrating a big win or thinking "I can do it" to build confidence.

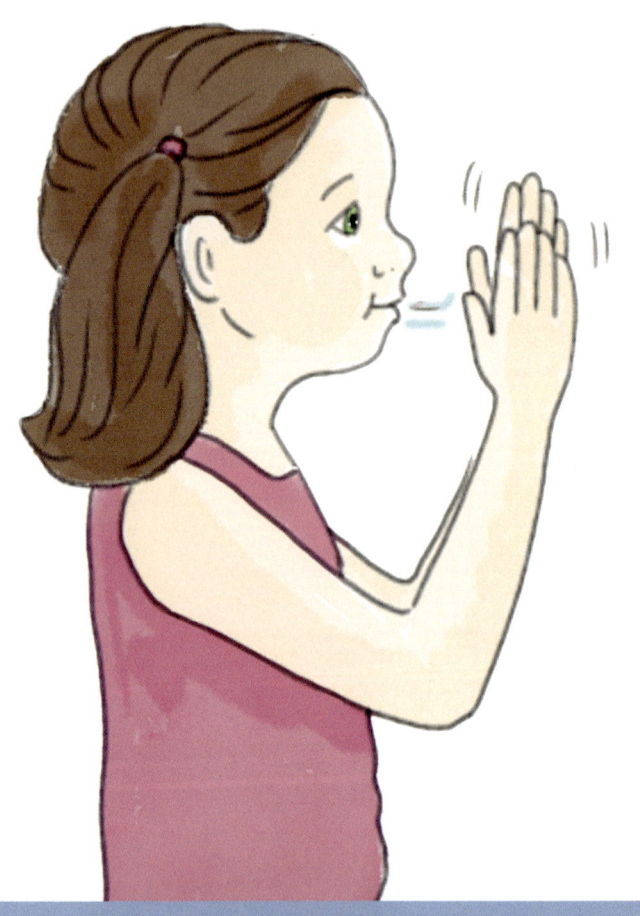

Rubbing Hands Breath

Rubbing Hands Breath

Bring your palms together in front of your heart center. Start to rub your palms together to generate heat. At the same time, bring your rubbing palms up to your mouth. Inhale deeply then exhale slowly while blowing your "fire" hands. Repeat the steps a few times.

> VARIATION: Cup your hands in front of your mouth and blow into your "fireplace."

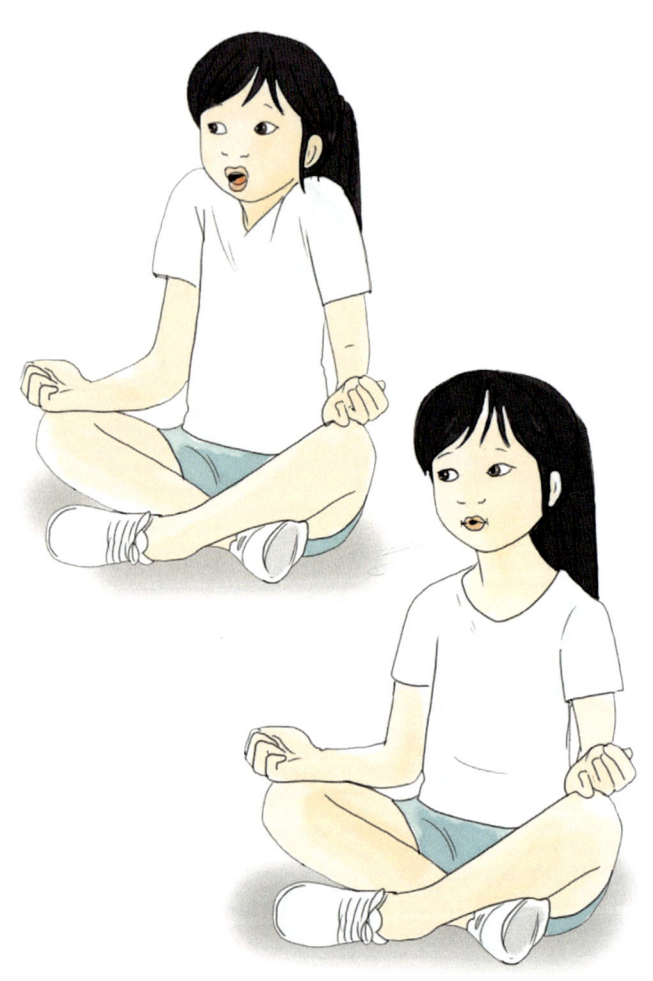

Shoulder Breath

Shoulder Breath

This is a great breath exercise to release tension from your shoulders, especially after you've been sitting at a desk for a period of time. Come to a comfortable sitting position and, if it's comfortable, close your eyes. On an inhale, raise your shoulders toward your ears. After a pause, exhale while releasing your shoulders back down. Repeat these steps as long as it feels comfortable.

> IMAGINE: Touching your shoulders to your eyes or that you're an elephant with big ears.

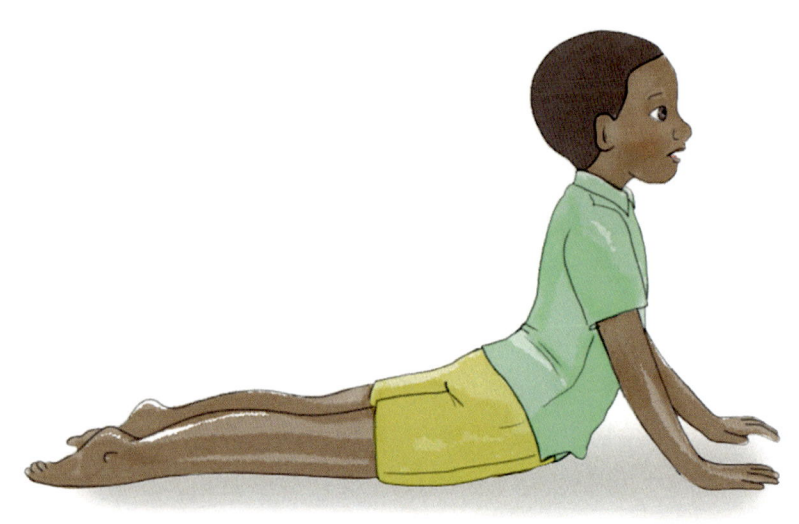

Snake Breath

Snake Breath

Lie on your tummy and place your palms flat next to your shoulders. Pressing into your hands, lift your head and shoulders off the ground. Take in a deep breath and exhale with a "hissing" sound like a snake.

> VARIATION: Stay seated while "hissing" like a snake.

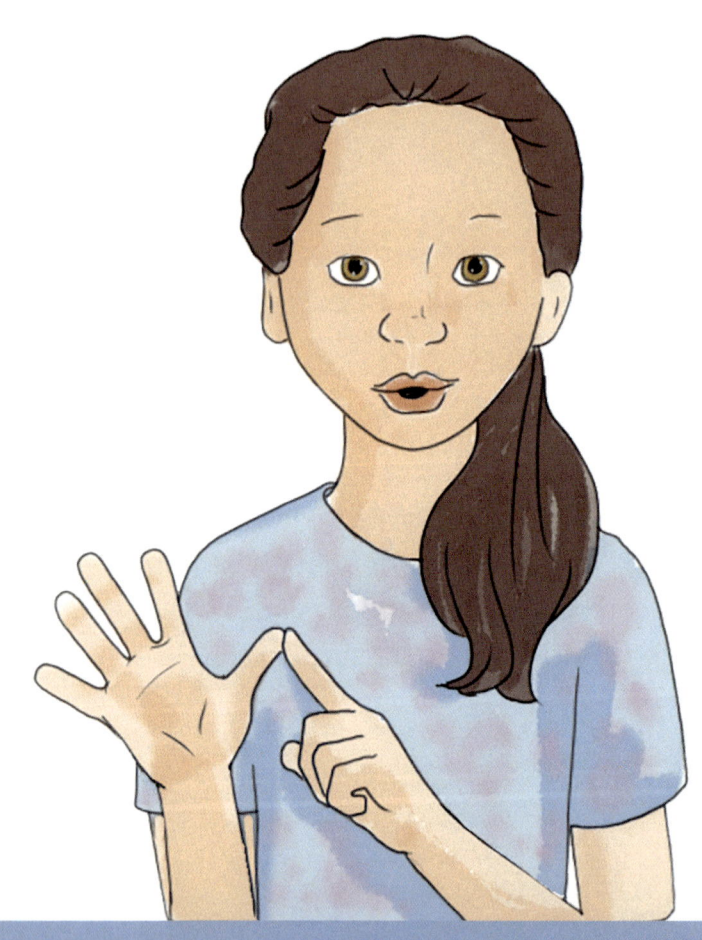

Take 5 Breath

Take 5 Breath

Take your right hand and spread your fingers like a star. Place your left pointer finger at the base of your right pinky finger. As you take a deep inhale, slide your pointer finger up your pinky finger. Pause briefly at the top of the finger. Then exhale fully while tracing the inside of your pinky finger. Repeat the inhale up your ring finger and exhale down your ring finger. Continue tracing your fingers and matching to your breath until you come to the outside of your thumb after five deep inhales and exhales. You can also trace your left hand if that's more comfortable.

> IMAGINE: Your pointer finger is going up and down a rollercoaster ride at a fun park.

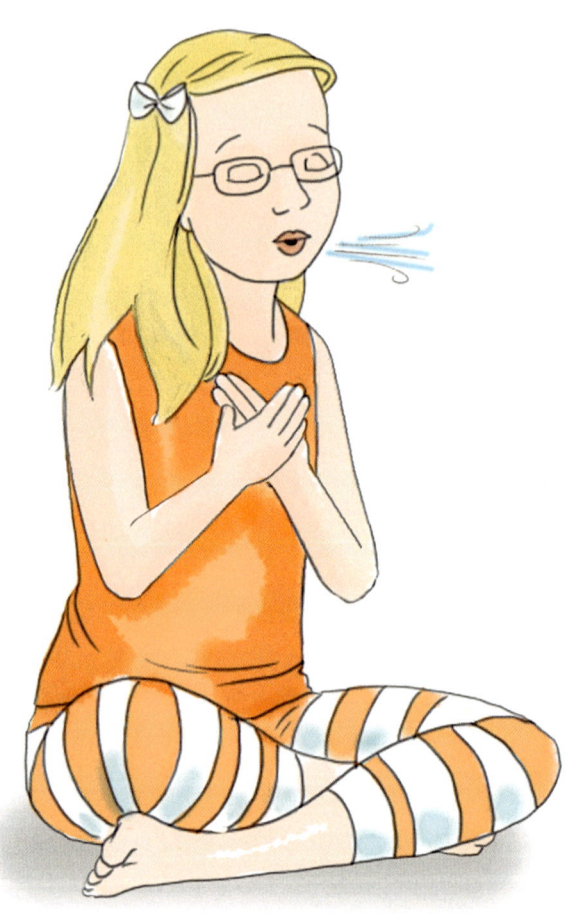

Three Deep Breaths

Three Deep Breaths

Cross your palms on your chest. Take a moment to feel the rise and fall of your breath. Close your eyes, if that's comfortable. Then take a deep inhale for three counts through your nose and exhale audibly through your mouth for three counts (or longer). Repeat these steps three times before going back to breathing naturally.

> VARIATION: Instead of the audible exhale, try creating an "om" sound.

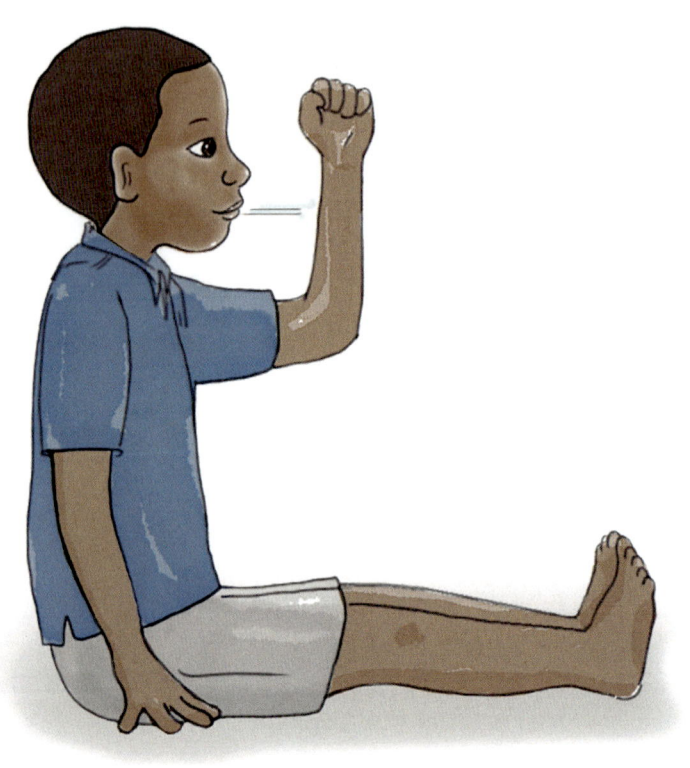

Truck Driver Breath

Truck Driver Breath

Come to sitting in an L position in a Staff Pose or sitting upright in a chair. Raise one hand, pretending to be a truck driver blowing the horn. Inhale deeply through your nose. Then exhale with your mouth open, making the sound of a truck horn: "Ah, ahhh." Repeat the steps to make more truck horn sounds. You could also cover your ears to intensify the sound of the truck horn.

> VARIATION: Pretend to be an engineer sounding a train horn.

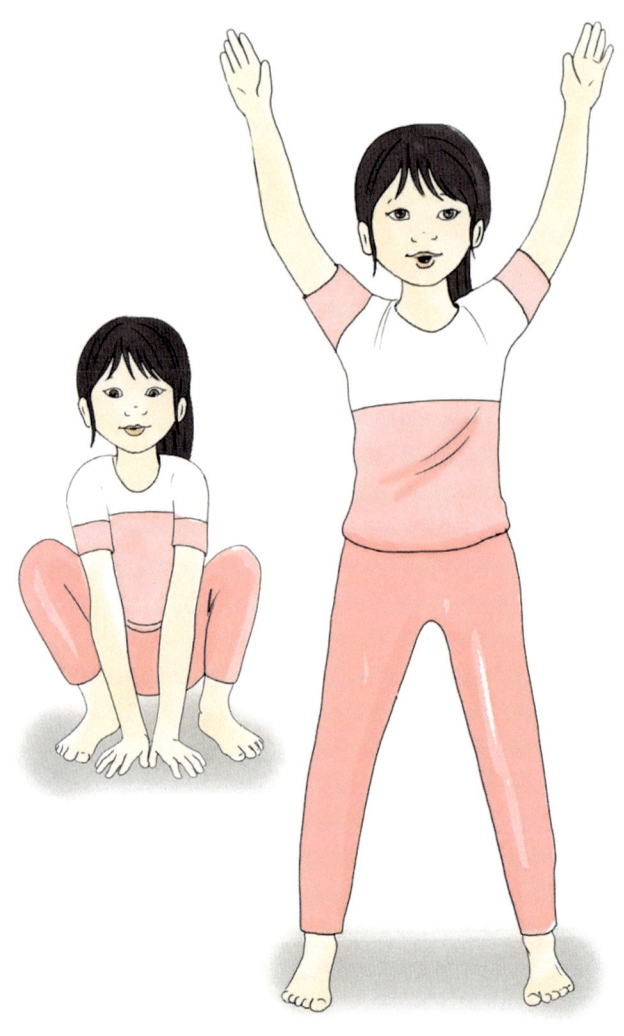

Volcano Breath

Volcano Breath

Come to a squat position with your hands on the ground between your legs. On a deep inhale, come to a standing position with your arms straight up above you as if you are an exploding volcano. Pause briefly at the top of the inhale (with your arms up), then exhale slowly, bring your arms down, and come back to the squat position. Repeat the steps a few times, pretending to be an erupting volcano.

> VARIATIONS: Be a seed growing into a tree or a frog jumping up to catch a fly.

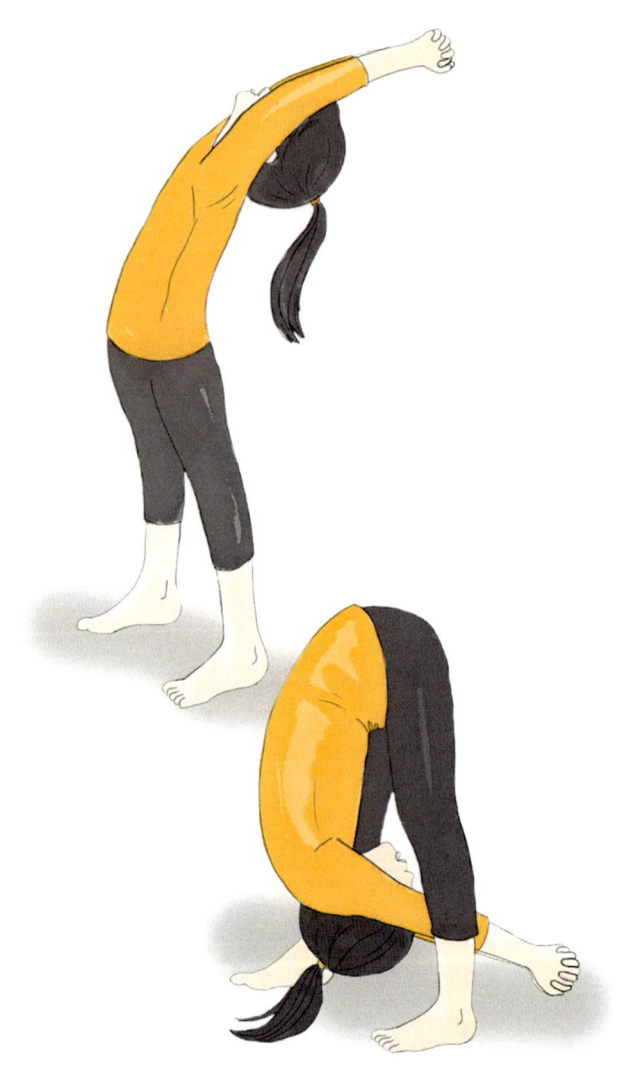

Woodchopper Breath

Woodchopper Breath

Stand tall in Mountain Pose and take a few deep breaths. Step your feet out a little wider than hip-width apart. Clasp your hands in front of your body. Take a long breath in while raising your hands above your head. On a vigorous exhale with your mouth open, forcefully take your hands down between your legs. Hang your head and completely let go of all the tension in your body. Close your eyes, if that feels comfortable. Repeat the steps, pretending to be a woodchopper cutting a log for a campfire. Repeat this technique a few times, allowing the children to find their own rhythm. Stand tall in Mountain Pose again and come back to breathing naturally. Let the children feel the effects of this energizing breath technique.

> VARIATION: Be an elephant drinking from a lake.

Breathing Exercise GAMES

On the following pages you'll find three breathing card games to spark your imagination, using our *Breathing Exercise Cards for Kids*. Also, you can encourage your children to make up their own games to learn the breathing exercises.

1. Play a Breathing Cards Dice Game

How to play a dice game with breathing cards for kids:

1. Grab a die from a board game you have at home.

2. Write the numbers 1 through 6 on sticky notes, one note for each number. You can write both the numeral and the number symbol found on dice.

3. Have your child pick out six breathing cards from the deck.

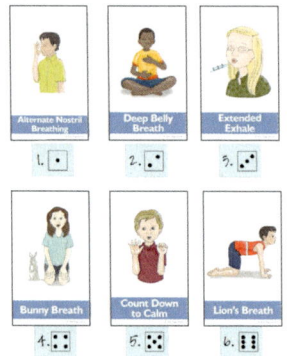

4. Stick a number note on each breathing card.

5. Roll the die and practice the breathing exercise associated with that number.

You could use a large die if working with a large group of kids. This simple dice yoga game would be great to bring traveling with you because all you need is a set of dice and breathing cards. Your child can easily change up the game by simply sticking the numbered sticky notes on different cards.

2. Play a Breathing Exercise Memory Game

Here's how to play the Breathing Exercise Memory Game:

1. The first person does a breathing exercise.

2. The second person does that first breathing exercise and then adds another breathing exercise to the sequence.

3. The first person then does the first two breaths and adds another breathing exercise.

4. Play continues as long as you like!

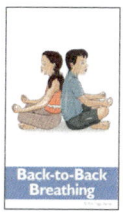 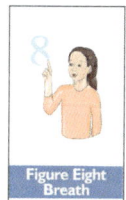 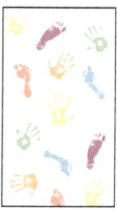 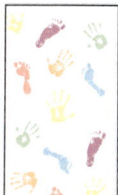

3. Play a Breathing Exercise Spinner Game

Here's how to play a Breathing Exercise Spinner Game:

1. Grab a deck of breathing exercise cards.

2. Place a Post-it note under one corner of a fidget spinner (or any other kind of spinner) to act as a pointer.

3. Pick out six breathing exercise cards and arrange them in a circle around the spinner.

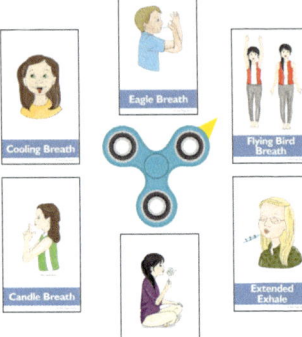

4. You might want to use Blu Tack or something similar on the bottom of the spinner to make sure it doesn't spin away.

5. Spin the spinner and then practice the breathing exercise that the pointer lands on.

You can change the breathing exercise cards after a few rounds and play again!

For even more ideas for how to play with yoga cards for kids, visit the Kids Yoga Stories website:
www.kidsyogastories.com/yoga-cards-for-kids-games/

About Kids Yoga Stories

We hope you enjoyed your Kids Yoga Stories experience. Visit WWW.KIDSYOGASTORIES.COM to:

RECEIVE UPDATES. For yoga tips, updates, giveaways, articles, kids yoga sequences, and activity ideas, sign up for our free Kids Yoga Stories Newsletter.

CONNECT WITH US. Please share with us about your yoga experiences. Send pictures of yourself practicing the poses. Describe your yoga journey on our social media pages (Facebook, Pinterest, Twitter, Instagram, and Google+).

CHECK OUT FREE STUFF. Read our articles on books, yoga, parenting, and travel. Check out our free kids yoga resources and coloring pages.

READ OR WRITE A REVIEW. Read what others have to say about our yoga books and kids yoga lesson plans. Post your own review on Amazon or on our website. We would love to hear how you enjoyed these monthly yoga ideas.

Thank you for your support in spreading our message of integrating learning, movement, and fun.

Giselle
KIDS YOGA STORIES
www.kidsyogastories.com
www.facebook.com/kidsyogastories
www.pinterest.com/kidsyogastories
www.twitter.com/kidsyogastories
www.amazon.com/author/giselleshardlow
www.plus.google.com/+giselleshardlow
www.goodreads.com/giselleshardlow

About the Author

GISELLE SHARDLOW draws from her experiences as a teacher, traveler, mother, and yogi to write her yoga stories for kids. The purpose of her yoga books is to foster happy, healthy, and globally educated children. She lives in Boston with her husband and daughter.

About the Illustrator

VALERIE BOUTHYETTE is an award-winning graphic designer and fine artist, who holds degrees in Advertising Art and Design and is a NYS Certified Early Childhood teacher. Valerie calls on her imagination and memories of childhood to create illustrations that warm your heart and make you smile. She creates in her studio nestled in the farmlands, which she refers to as "her heaven." Valerie lives with her husband in upstate NY, where they also own a small horse boarding facility.

Yoga Books by Giselle Shardlow

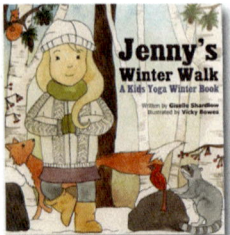
Jenny's Winter Walk

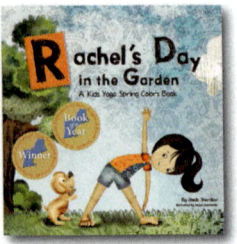
Rachel's Day in the Garden

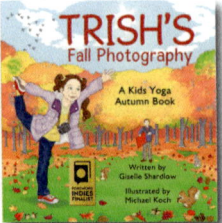
Trish's Fall Photography

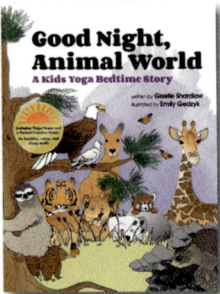
Good Night, Animal World

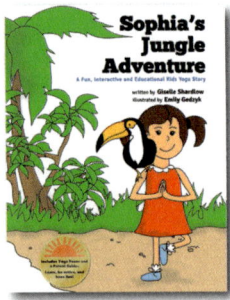
Sophia's Jungle Adventure

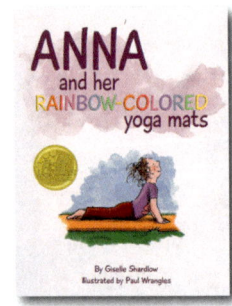
Anna and her Rainbow-Colored Yoga Mats

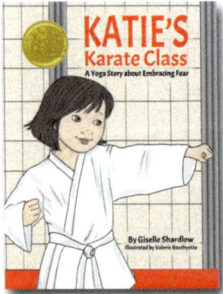
Katie's Karate Class

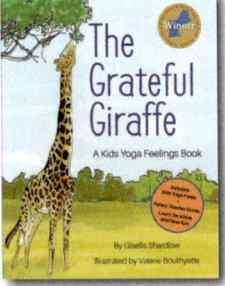
The Grateful Giraffe

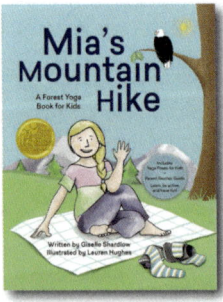
Mia's Mountain Hike

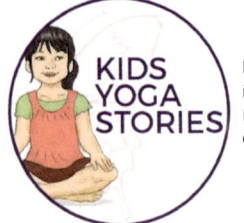

Many of the books above are available
in Spanish and eBook format.
Buy now at www.amazon.com/author/giselleshardlow
OR www.KidsYogaStories.com/store

Made in the USA
San Bernardino, CA
18 February 2020